TRYPOPHOBIA

DR MIRIAM KINAI

ISBN: 1492171433

ISBN-13: 978-1492171430

CONTENTS

DR MIRIAM KINAI

1

WHAT IS
TRYPOPHOBIA?

Trypophobia is the intense and irrational fear of small holes which can be clustered either symmetrically or asymmetrically.

These fear inducing tiny holes can include:

1. Enlarged skin pores

2. Bone marrow

3. Teeth cavities

4. Swiss cheese

5. Lotus seed pods

6. Cantaloupe, pumpkin, squash

7. Crumpets

8. Honeycomb

9. Corn cobs without the corn

10. Pumice

11. Coral

12. Sponges

* * * * *

2

WHAT CAUSES TRYPOPHOBIA?

The exact cause of trypophobia is unknown.

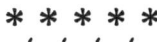

3

WHAT ARE THE SYMPTOMS OF TRYPOPHOBIA?

Symptoms of trypophobia include experiencing the following on seeing many small holes:

1. General body discomfort

2. Itchy sensations

3. Developing goose bumps and feeling like your skin is crawling

4. Feeling anxious and nervous

5. Developing nausea and vomiting

6. Developing panic attacks with sweating, shaking, palpitations or irregular heartbeats and shortness of breath.

7. Fearing that the tiny holes will grow into large holes in which they may fall and disappear

8. Some tryphobics fear tiny clustered holes but are unable to look away

* * * * *

4

WHAT IS THE TREATMENT FOR TRYPOPHOBIA?

The treatment for trypophobia includes:

1. Behavior Therapy

Trypophobics are taught how to change and eradicate unwanted behaviors when they are exposed to numerous tiny holes.

***

2. Cognitive Therapy

Trypophobes are taught how to change their thinking patterns when they are exposed to clusters of tiny holes so that they can have different reaction patterns.

3. Cognitive Behavioral Therapy (CBT)

CBT is a combination of Behavior Therapy and Cognitive Therapy.

***

4. Systemic Desensitization

The first step is to learn an effective relaxation technique like abdominal breathing so that you can manage the distress you experience when facing the phobia.

Abdominal or diaphragmatic breathing simply involves inhaling deeply through your nose until your abdomen rises, holding your breath for a few moments and then exhaling completely through your nose until your abdomen falls.

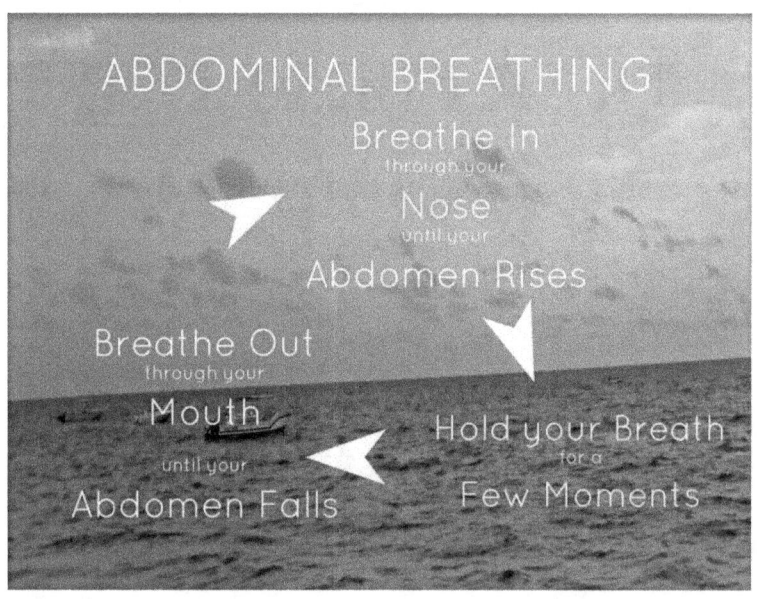

The second step of systemic desensitization involves imagining yourself looking at tiny clustered holes.

Therefore, imagine yourself looking at the least scary image of tiny clustered holes and take several deep breaths to reduce the distress of that imagination. For example this might be a block of Swiss cheese for you though it varies from one person to another.

Once you can comfortably imagine yourself looking at that image, imagine yourself looking at a more scary image of tinnier clustered holes. For example this might be looking at a honeycomb. Use abdominal breathing or any other relaxation technique to counter the distress of your imagination until you are comfortable seeing yourself looking at many honeycombs.

Continue visualizing yourself looking at progressively scarier images of tinnier clustered holes until you are able to visualize yourself looking at enlarged skin pores since the tinniest holes and those on human skin are said to be the scariest.

At each phase ensure that you use abdominal breathing to counter the stress of your imagination until you can eventually look at those holes with your physical eyes without getting distressed.

If you develop difficulties, consult a professional so that they can help you with this process of systemic desensitization.

***

5. Bible Therapy

a. The first Bible therapy principle for fear intervention is to ask God to help you overcome trypophobia. As you pray, use Scriptures since the Word of God is the Sword of the Spirit (Ephesians 6:17) that God has given us to fight with.

Scriptures that you can pray to overcome trypophobia include:

i. Father God, I ask you in the name of Jesus to help me overcome this fear of tiny clustered holes since You have not given me a spirit of fear but You have given me a spirit of power and of love and a sound mind. (Adapted 2 Timothy 1:7)

ii. Father God I ask You in the name of Jesus to help me remember that You are my helper and therefore I should not fear tiny clustered holes. (Adapted Hebrews 13:6)

iii. I say to you Lord, "You are my refuge and my fortress, My God in You I trust.

Surely You shall deliver me from this fear of clustered tiny holes.

You cover me with Your feathers and under Your wings I take refuge.

Your truth shall be my surrounding shield.

I shall not be afraid of tiny holes during the day or during the night.

I shall not be afraid of looking at holes of any size in the dark and where there is light.

A thousand people may be harmed by trypophobia but it shall not harm me.

Because I have made You Lord my refuge, and You the Most High God, my dwelling place, no evil from fearing holes shall befall me and this trypophobia shall not come to my home.

You God have put Your angels in charge of me to protect me in all my ways and in their hands they shall bear me up so that I do not hurt my mind.

I shall crush this fear of clustered tiny holes under my foot.

Because I have set my love upon You, You will deliver me from trypophobia. You will set me on high because I know Your name.

I will call on You and You will answer me. You will be with me when I face this challenge of holes.

You will deliver me from trypophobia and honor me." (Adapted Psalm 91)

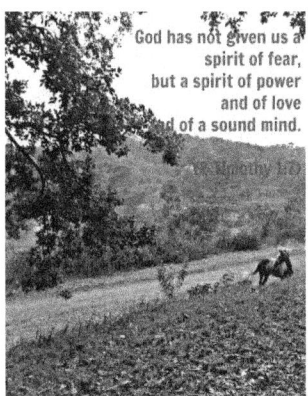

b. The second Bible therapy principle is to put on the helmet of salvation since it is part of the armor of God that we need to put on to fight our spiritual battles. (Ephesians 6:14-17)

All you need to put on this helmet of salvation is to say with your mouth that "Jesus is Lord" and believe in your heart that God raised Him from the dead when He died for our sins and you will be saved. (Romans 10:9)

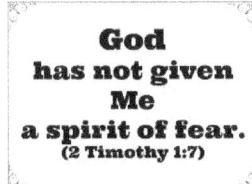

c. The third Bible therapy fear intervention is to remove all fearful thoughts from your mind so that you can **Be renewed in the spirit of your mind.** (Ephesians 4:23) To do this, meditate on awesome Bible verses like the following to help you overcome this phobia:

i. (*Insert your name***) be strong and courageous. I am not afraid of tiny clustered holes because the Lord my God is the One who goes with me and He will never leave me nor forsake me.** (Adapted Deuteronomy 31:6)

ii. God has not given me a spirit of fearing tiny clustered holes. He has given me a spirit of power and of love and a sound mind. (Adapted 2 Timothy 1:7)

Memorize these Scriptures and carry them in your mind or write them down on a piece of paper and read them when you encounter a frightening situation.

In addition, decide to believe these Scriptures since having faith in God and in His Word is how you hold up your shield of faith which is another of our spiritual warfare weapons and the weapon that is able to quench all the fiery darts of the enemy. (Ephesians 6:16)

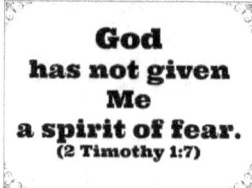

God has not given Me a spirit of fear. (2 Timothy 1:7)

d. The fourth Bible therapy principle is to read at least one chapter of the Bible everyday because the Gospel is another of our warfare weapons and so that you can learn more fear fighting Scriptures to meditate on.

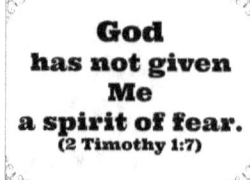

God has not given Me a spirit of fear. (2 Timothy 1:7)

e. The fifth Bible therapy principle is to speak the Word of God over your mind because it is the sword of the Spirit that we are to wield to fight our spiritual battles. Positive Christian affirmations that you can confess include:

i. Though I see many tiny clustered holes, I will not fear because God is with me. (Adapted Psalm 23:4)

ii. I will trust and not be afraid of tiny holes because the Lord is my strength. (Adapted Isaiah 12:2)

iii. The Lord is my helper and I will not fear tiny clustered holes. (Adapted Hebrews 13:6)

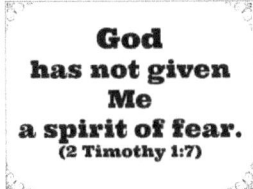

f. The sixth Bible therapy principle is to live right. Be righteous and truthful in all your dealings because the breastplate of righteousness and the belt of truth and are the other parts of the armor of God that we need to put on to fight our spiritual battles. (Ephesians 6:14-17)

###

ABOUT THE AUTHOR

Dr. Miriam Kinai is a medical doctor and a certified clinical aromatherapy practitioner.

You can visit her blog at http://www.MyBlogBookClub.com or follow her on twitter at http://twitter.com/AlmasiHealth

Email enquiries to almasihealthcare@yahoo.com with BOOKS as your subject.

SIMPLIFIED MEDICINE

Simplified Medicine uses plain and easy to understand English to teach you about the causes, risk factors, symptoms, tests, treatment, prognosis and prevention of numerous diseases like:

* Bile Duct Cancer

* Osteosarcoma (Bone Cancer)

* Throat Cancer

* Congestive Heart Failure

* Legionnaire's Disease

* West Nile Virus

* Cryptosporidiosis

* Cyclospora

* Polymyalgia Rheumatica

* Sarcoidosis

* Alcoholic liver cirrhosis

* Dry Drowning

* Prosopagnosia

*****

USMLE 1 & 2 QUESTIONS & ANSWERS

USMLE 1 & 2 Questions & Answers is filled with high yield questions with detailed answers and color pictures of medical conditions to help you prepare and pass your professional medical examinations.

These revision questions cover the following subspecialities:

* Cardiology

* Dermatology

* Embryology

* Emergency Medicine

* Endocrinology

* Gastroenterology

* Gynecology

* Neurology

* Oncology

* Pulmonolgy

* Rheumatology

*****

HERBS AND SPICES FOR THE COOK, HEALER AND BEAUTICIAN

Herbs and Spices for the Cook, Healer and Beautician uses color pictures and clear explanations to teach you about more than 70 healing herbs and spices.

You will learn about their:

* Therapeutic (healing) uses

* Drug interactions

* Contraindications (when not to use them)

* Cooking tips

* Beauty tips

*****

INTERNATIONAL GOURMET HERB AND SPICE BLENDS

International Gourmet Herb and Spice Blends teaches you how to prepare exotic herb and spice blends from around the world. You will discover the recipes for:

* Barbecue Rub, Cajun, Apple Pie and Pumpkin Pie Spice Mixes from America

* Pudding Spice Mix from Britain

* 5 Spice Mix from China

* Berbere Spice Mix from Ethiopia

* Curry Powder and Garam Masala from India

* Bouquet Garni, Herbs de Provence and Quatre Epices from France

* Herb Mix from Italy

* Jerk Seasoning from Jamaica

* Shichimi Togarashi from Japan

* Pilau Spice Blend from Kenya

* Chili Powder from Mexico

* Baharat Spice Blend from the Middle East

* Ras El Hanout from Morocco

*****

THE QUICK GOURMET CHEF

The Quick Gourmet is an essential culinary skills cookbook which teaches how to make simple, divine dishes.

You will learn how to make:

* Hot Chocolate Mixes and Drinks

* Hot Chai Tea Mixes and Drinks

* Hot Coffee Mixes and Drinks

* Sensational Smoothies

* Non-Dairy Smoothies

* Chocolate Covered Strawberries

* Chocolate Truffles

* Healthy Chicken Salads

* Healthy Tuna Salads

* Savory Salsas

* Herb Butter

* Cheese Dips and Sauces

* Gourmet Sandwiches

* Perfect Hard Boiled Eggs

* A Cheese Board

* Natural Food Color

*****

HOW TO STYLE AND PHOTOGRAPH FOOD

Regardless of whether you are an aspiring food blogger or you want to make money online selling stock photos, How To Style and Photograph Food, uses color pictures and clear explanations to teach you the food photography tips that can help you improve your digital camera photography skills so that you can begin photographing food like a pro.

You will learn:

* The equipment that you need

* How to set up the lighting

* How to prepare the stage

* How to style the food

* How to shoot the food

*****

HOW TO MAKE NATURAL SKIN CARE PRODUCTS SERIES

Books in this series include:

* How to Make Natural Bath and Body Oils

* How to Make Natural Bath bombs

* How to Make Natural Bath melts

* How to Make Natural Bath milks

* How to Make Natural Bath salts

* How to Make Natural Bath teas

* How to Make Natural Body butters

* How to Make Natural Body lotions

* How to Make Natural Body scrubs

* How to Make Natural Face Scrubs

* How to Make Natural Herb infused oils

* How to Make Natural Massage bars

* How to Make Natural Soap

* How to Make Natural Solid and Liquid Castile Soap

* How to Make Natural Solid and Liquid Perfumes

* How to Make Natural Sunscreen Lotions

* How to Make Natural Toothpaste and Tooth Whitening Powder

* How to Make Ubtan Powder

*****

THE ESSENTIALS OF AROMATHERAPY ESSENTIAL OILS

The Essentials of Aromatherapy Essential Oils by Dr Miriam Kinai teaches you how to use aromatherapy oils to improve your physical, mental and emotional well being.

The author's experience as a medical doctor and clinical aromatherapy practitioner have enabled her to write a highly informative guide for those who want to utilize the healing benefits of these natural plant essences.

You will discover:

* The safety information and therapeutic uses of 18 essential oils

* How to blend essential oils

* The characteristics and uses of 14 carrier oils

* How to Dilute Essential Oils with Carrier Oils

* How to Use Essential Oils

* Cautionary Measures when using Essential Oils

* Numerous Essential Oil Recipes for bath products as well as skin care and hair care products

The Essentials of Aromatherapy Essential Oils will leave you with a clear understanding of how you can safely use aromatherapy essential oils to heal yourself naturally.

*****

MEDICAL AROMATHERAPY FOR HEALTH PROFESSIONALS

Medical Aromatherapy for Healthcare Professionals by Dr Miriam Kinai teaches you how to use essential oils to treat physical diseases and emotional disorders.

The author's experience as a medical doctor and clinical aromatherapy practitioner have enabled her to write a highly informative guide for those who want to utilize the healing benefits of these natural plant essences.

You will discover how to use essential oils to:

* Treat skin diseases like acne, eczema and psoriasis

* Treat other physical diseases like high blood pressure, arthritis, coughs and colds

* Manage mental and emotional conditions like anxiety, depression, anger and stress

* Relieve the symptoms of menopause and premenstrual tension

* Lessen insomnia and impotence

Medical Aromatherapy for Healthcare Professionals is therefore an essential resource for holistic healthcare practitioners like massage therapists, naturopaths and herbalists.

It is also a useful resource for conventional medicine healthcare providers like physicians and nurses who want to begin practicing integrative medicine and for patients who want to improve their health naturally by using aromatherapy oils.

*****

AROMATHERAPY COURSE

Aromatherapy Course by Dr Miriam Kinai tutors you on how to use essential oils to improve your physical, mental and emotional well being.

The author's experience as a medical doctor and clinical aromatherapy practitioner have enabled her to create a highly informative course on how to use these natural plant essences.

You will learn:

* The safety information and therapeutic uses of essential oils like clary sage, eucalyptus, geranium, grapefruit, lavender, lemon, lemongrass, marjoram, orange (sweet), patchouli, peppermint, Roman chamomile, rose, rosemary, sandalwood, spearmint, tea tree and ylang ylang.

* The safety information and therapeutic uses of carrier oils like apricot kernel oil, avocado oil, borage seed oil, calendula oil, carrot seed oil, castor oil, evening primrose oil, fractionated coconut oil, jojoba, olive oil, rosehip oil, sunflower oil, sweet almond oil and virgin coconut oil.

* How to blend essential oils

* How to dilute essential oils with carrier oils

* How to administer essential oils

* How to make natural healing products from numerous aromatherapy recipes

* How to utilize the healing benefits of essentials oils even if you do not have prior training in aromatherapy

The Aromatherapy Course will leave you with a clear understanding of how you can heal yourself and your family naturally by using essentials oils on your body and in your home.

*****

DEALING WITH DEPRESSION NATURALLY

Dealing with Depression Naturally presents a holistic approach to managing depression with natural antidepressants. You will learn how to treat depression with:

* Aromatherapy

* Art therapy

* Christian Biblical principles

* Chromotherapy

* Diet therapy

* Eco-therapy

* Herbal therapy

* Home decor therapy

* Music therapy

* Phototherapy

* Exercise therapy

* Self-Psychotherapy

* Social therapy

* Talk therapy

* Vitamin therapy

* Writing therapy

*****

CHRISTIAN LIFE COACHING HANDBOOK

Christian Life Coaching Handbook offers a Biblical approach to managing different aspects of life.

You will learn:

* Christian anger management

* Christian conflict resolution

* Christian depression treatment

* Christian goal setting

* Christian marital stress management

* Christian stress management

* How to assert yourself

* How to defeat fear

* How to love yourself

* How to overcome shyness

* How to resist temptation

* How to stop being a people pleaser

*****

CHRISTIAN SPIRITUAL WARFARE

Christian Spiritual Warfare teaches you the awesome Bible verses you can use as spiritual warfare prayers, Christian affirmations and in your Christian meditation sessions as you fight your spiritual battles.

You will learn how to fight for the following with Bible verses:

* Marriage * Children * Health

* Christian Faith * Christian Ministry

* Country

* Finances * Job * Business

* Peace of Mind * Restoration * Self Esteem * Self Love

You will also learn how to fight against the following with Bible verses:

* Addiction * Temptation

* Being Single * Infertility

* Opposition * Oppression

* Worry * Fear

* Feelings of Condemnation * Confusion

* Danger * Death * Despair * Discouragement

* Impatience * Insomnia * Laziness * Loneliness

* Poverty * Pride * Sadness

* Vengeance * Weakness

* A Foul Mouth * Lying

*****

27

DARK SKIN DERMATOLOGY COLOR ATLAS

Dark Skin Dermatology Color Atlas is filled with clear explanations and color photos of skin, hair, and nail diseases affecting people with skin of color or Fitzpatrick skin types IV, V, and VI.

Topics covered include Acne Vulgaris, Alopecia Areata, Anal Warts, Angioedema, Aphthous Ulcers, Atopic Dermatitis, Blastomycosis, Blister Beetle Dermatitis or Nairobi Fly Dermatitis, Cellulitis, Chronic Ulcers, Confetti Hypopigmentation, Cutaneous T Cell Lymphoma, Cutaneous Tuberculosis, Dermatitis Artefacta, Erythema Nodosum,

Exfoliative Erythroderma, Gianotti Crosti Syndrome, Hand Dermatitis, Hemangioma, Herpes Zoster, Ichthyosis, Ingrown Toenails, Irritant Contact Dermatitis, Kaposi Sarcoma, Keloids, Keratoderma Blenorrhagica, Klippel Trenaunay Weber Syndrome, Leishmaniasis, Leprosy, Leukonychia, Lichen Nitidus, Lichen Planus,

Lichenoid Drug Eruption, Linear Epidermal Nevus, Linear IgA Dermatosis (LAD), Lipodermatosclerosis, Lymphangioma Circumscriptum, Miliaria, Molluscum Contagiosum, Neurofibromatosis, Nickel Dermatitis, Onychomadesis, Onychomycosis, Palmoplantar Eccrine Hidradenitis, Papular Pruritic Eruption (PPE), Paronychia, Pellagra, Pemphigus Foliaceous,

Pemphigus Vulgaris, Piebaldism, Pityriasis Rosea, Pityriasis Rubra Pilaris, Plantar Hyperkeratosis, Plantar Warts, Poikiloderma, Postinflammatory Hyperpigmentation and Hypopigmentation, Post Topical Steroids Hypopigmentation, Psoriasis, Pyogenic Granuloma or Lobular Capillary Hemangioma, Scabies, Seborrheic Dermatitis, Steven Johnson Syndrome (SJS) and Toxic Epidermal Necrolysis (TEN),

Sunburn, Systemic Sclerosis, Tinea Capitis, Tinea Pedis, Tinea Versicolor, Traction Alopecia, Urticaria, Vasculitis, Vitiligo, and Xanthelasma.

*****